40 Healthy Habits for a Better You

Table of Contents

Summary

Healthy living is not a new "craze" or "fad". It's timeless wisdom to help you live the best life that you can, whether you're five or 85. And it's never too late to start making changes, even small ones, which can help you to begin living a better life and feel better spiritually, physically and mentally.

This book is designed to give you "snippets" of ways to live a better life. Many of the ideas you may already be familiar with, while some may be totally new. We hope you find it as useful and thought provoking to read as we did to write!

Chapter 1: Easy tips for making small changes.

"And suddenly you know: It's time to start something new and trust the magic of beginnings."
— Meister Eckhart

There is something refreshing about making a new start. The promise of something that has not yet begun, so it has not yet been thwarted. The possibilities are endless, and failure is not yet an option.

It's time to start at the beginning. To begin making small changes that can improve your health and your outlook on life. Here are our ten favorites, in no particular order, designed to give you a new start.

Start drinking...water, that is.

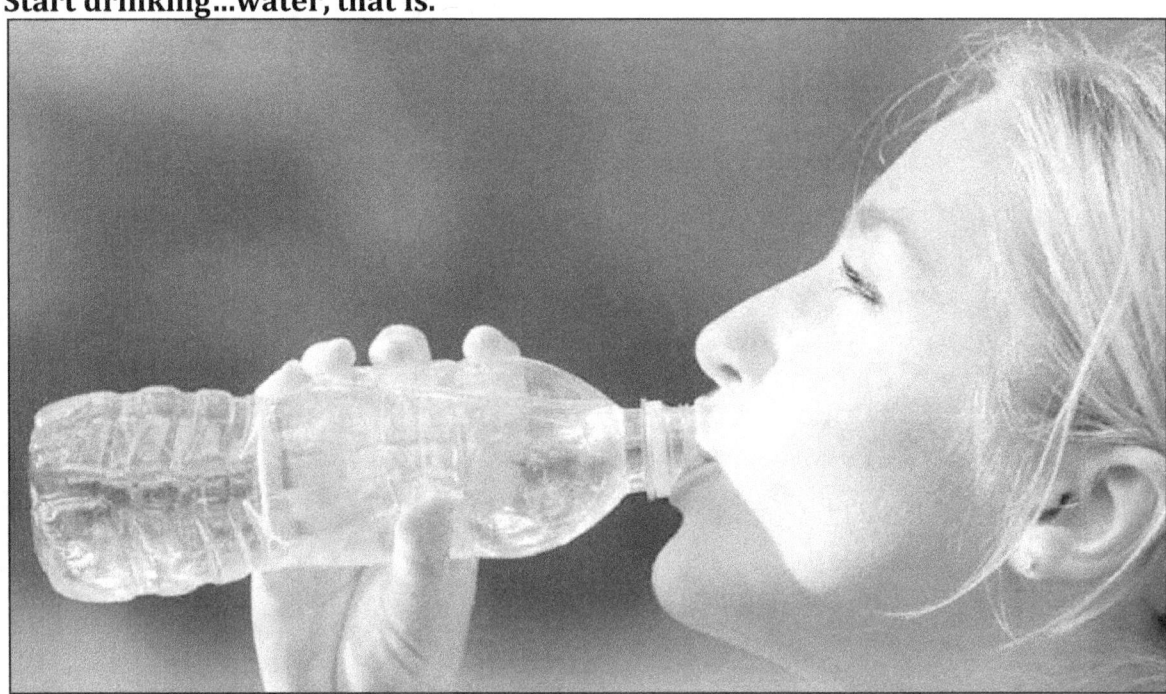

Most of us just simply don't drink enough water. We may drink a lot of other things...pop, juice, milk, coffee, tea...and while most of these things have water IN them, it's not the same thing. Drinking plain water is one of the easiest and most important things we can do.

- **It keeps you "balanced".** Your body is more than 60% water. Drinking enough water and keeping yourself properly hydrated helps your circulatory system to move nutrients around your body, keeps your temperature regulated and helps you to property digest your food.

- **It's great for your skin.** Skin that is properly hydrated looks and feels healthy. It helps to flush out toxins and is able to help reduce the risk of developing acne.
- **It keeps you "going"...literally!** Your kidneys work constantly to flush toxins out of your body, processing about 200 quarts of blood a day. Drinking enough water helps to flush the toxins, transporting urine to the bladder and eliminating them from your body.
- **It wakes you up.** One of the first symptoms of dehydration is fatigue. Drinking enough water keeps you hydrated, which means that your brain is able to focus on the task at hand...and you get more done!
- **It helps you lose weight.** Water helps you to feel full faster; meaning you eat less, meaning you start to lose weight...it's a win-win-win situation!

While how MUCH water you need to drink is up for debate, it is generally thought that adults need between 9 and 16 glasses of water a day. And if you think water is "blah", try one of the new water bottles with infusers in the middle and add cucumbers, berries, mint, herbs...whatever you need to perk it up. But whatever you do...start drinking!

Get up off that...couch.

Most of us just simply don't get enough exercise. And our sedentary lifestyle is taking its' toll on our health...physically AND mentally. In contrast to our ancestors, who spent much of their lives working...and working hard...our generation has become technology driven and permanently seated. And it's not good for us. Too much sitting can contribute to...

- Type 2 Diabetes.
- Heart Disease
- Obesity
- Arthritis

If you are used to sitting more than you're moving, it's probably best not to start with a PX90 workout routine. You could, however, start moving a little bit and work your way up. Try walking around the block, or up the street. Increase your distance a little bit every day, and try walking a little faster. Don't feel the need to be in a hurry—you are not competing against anyone but yourself.

If walking isn't your thing, try something you really enjoy. Put on your favorite music and dance around the living room. Buy a mini-trampoline and jump 'til you drop. Dig your kid's old jump rope out of the toy box and start skipping. The KIND of exercise isn't as important as just DOING something. And the benefits will make you glad you did!

Love the one you're with.

Spending time with the people that we love…and who love us back…is a great way to boost our health, both physical and mental. People who have strong social networks are generally happier not only with their social lives, but also with other aspects of their lives in general.

Spending time with friends and family is a fantastic way to get out of the house and on the move, boosting endorphins and improving our mental clarity and thought processes. And spending time with people who affirm us boosts our self-esteem, making us love ourselves (and them!) more.

Quit smoking. Right now. Immediately.

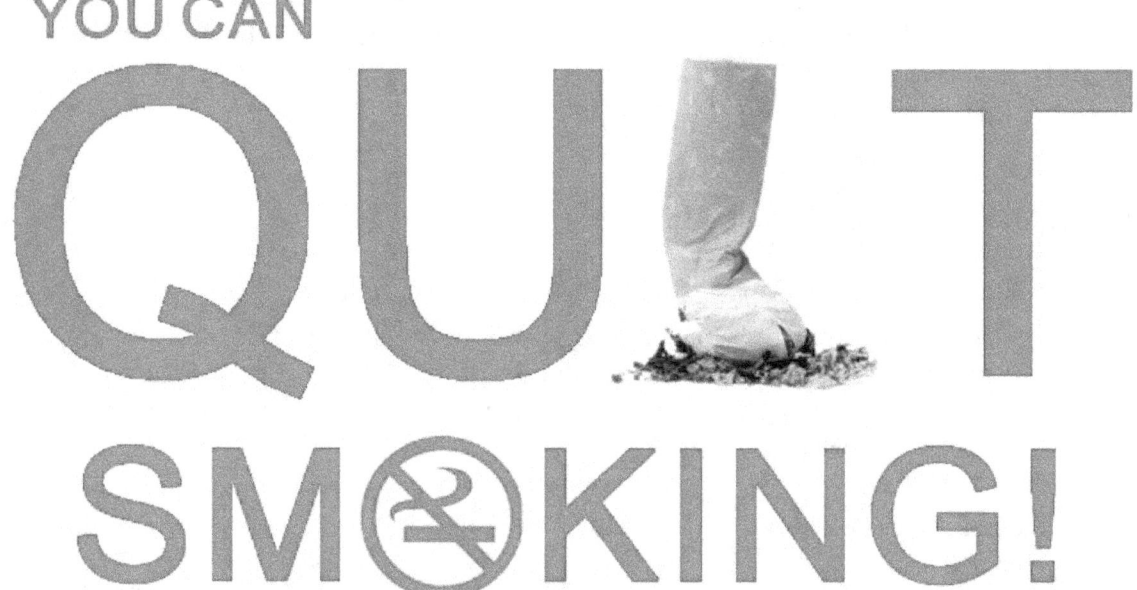

Smoking is one of the most dangerous habits you can have. It is the leading cause of lung cancer, causes COPD and can lead to heart disease. In addition, it makes your hair, clothes, car, breath, house and whatever else you touch smell, and it yellows your teeth. And it's ridiculously expensive.

Count your blessings…

There's an old children's Sunday School song that starts out "Count your blessings, name the one by one…" It's cute, and anyone who went through Sunday School between 1940 and now knows the song, but there is a nugget of truth to it.

By "counting your blessings", you are focusing on what you have, rather than what you don't. Your outlook on life will improve, and even if you don't have as much as the next guy, chances are you're doing pretty well. Even in our darkest days, there are things that we can count as blessings. Try keeping a "Blessing journal" and write down one thing every day that blessed your socks off. It doesn't have to be huge—it can be a beautiful sunset, a compliment or a particularly juicy blueberry. Just name something that made you realize, even for a second, how blessed you really are.

Volunteer.

Now that you're counting your own blessings, it's time to go be a blessing to someone else. Stepping outside of ourselves and making the world a little bit brighter for someone else is a great way to remind ourselves that we are not alone on this planet, and that we have the power to make a difference, even a small one, in someone else's life.

Use the sunscreen, Mabel.

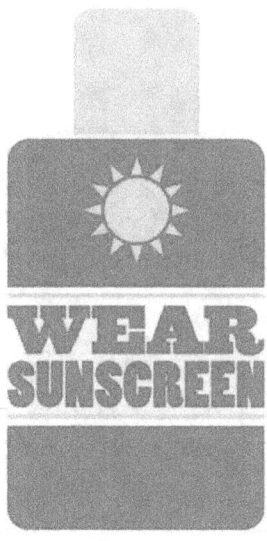

While we all wish we could get the "savage tan", the reality is that since we've killed off our ozone, the savage tan could literally kill us. That's because there is very little standing (or floating) in between us and the UV from the rays of the sun that cause skin damage.

At best, the UV rays age us and make us look old. And since they can cause melanoma, which is the deadliest form of skin cancer, getting that tan may shorten your life considerably. Dermatologists recommend using a sunscreen with an SPF of 15 or greater, and reapplying frequently as sweating and swimming can wash off your protection. If you have extremely fair skin, use a higher SPF and keep yourself covered if at all possible. You may not have that bikini body with the lifeguard tan, but on the positive side you'll still be alive. And don't even think about using a tanning bed. You might as well just go crawl into a microwave and cook yourself.

Eliminate the toxic people in your life.

We all have them—people that drag us down and make us feel like we're less than we are. Eliminating those people is hard, but doing so can boost your self-esteem and give you a healthier outlook on life. Toxic people can cause undue stress on our emotions, which puts stress on our body, which leads to depression and can be a contributing factor in auto-immune diseases such as Chronic Fatigue Syndrome and Fibromyalgia. Making yourself get rid of them can be just as stressful, but once it's done, you'll feel a whole lot better.

Sleep, baby, sleep.

Your body uses sleep to rest and repair itself. Studies have shown that people who get less than seven hours of sleep a night and more than nine hours a night are more prone to significant health problems than those who find their "sweet spot" and get between 7 & 9.

Sit up straight!

Slouching affects your health (it's hard on your spine, hips and neck) and believe it or not, it affects the way you feel about yourself. Sitting up a little straighter can be an instant confidence booster, making you feel better about yourself and projecting confidence to those around you. Your mom and your third grade teacher were right---sit up straight!

Now that we've given you some general tips for living a healthier lifestyle, let's break it down. The next few chapters will give you specific tips for a specific area of your life. Remember—we are just here to advise you—you'll have to do the work yourself!

Chapter 2: Change the way you eat.

Making small changes in the way that you eat can make a big difference in how you look and feel. While it is true that sometimes big changes are needed, starting small will give you the chance to adjust both mentally and physically, and you can work your way up to major changes gradually. Some easy ways to begin are...

Cut out the soda.

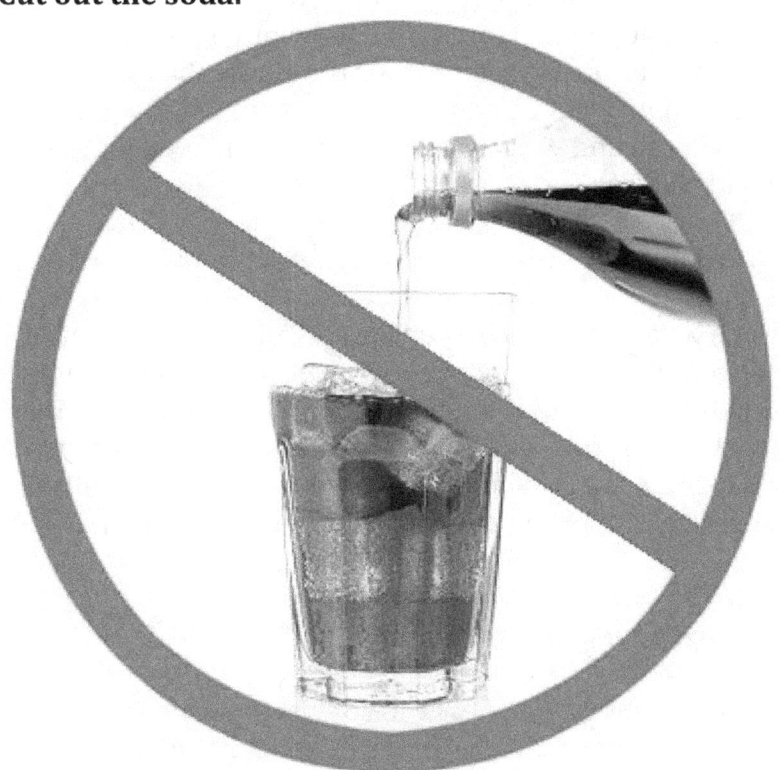

Soda has absolutely no nutritional benefits. It is loaded with high fructose corn syrup, which is slowly killing you, and it packs on way too many calories without providing any nutrition. And diet soda is worse. Artificial sweeteners have been proven to make you overeat, mess with your hormones, trick your taste buds, increase your risk of diabetes and pollute the water table. And if you have an autoimmune disease such as Fibromyalgia, artificial sweeteners exacerbate your symptoms, especially your pain level. Drink water instead. If you need that "kick" that soda gives you, try squeezing a lemon into your water, or drinking mineral water with lemon.

Plan your meals in advance.

Making a meal plan for the week helps you to avoid the "forgot to thaw something out so we'll just eat at a restaurant or order in" syndrome. It also keeps your food bills lower, since you aren't shopping for food you don't eat and then heading to a restaurant when you can't decide what to make for dinner. Even a simple plan, such as deciding what the main dish will be each night and then filling in around the edges with what you have on hand can make a big difference in your family's eating habits.

Make a list for the grocery store.

Going to the grocery store without a list (and especially if you don't have a list AND you're hungry) almost guarantees that you will forget half of what you need, spend too much money and come out without the ingredients for the meals that you plan to make. Taking a few minutes to look over your kitchen, figure out what you've already got that you can use that week and writing down what you'll need will save you time, money, frustration and calories.

Shop the perimeter of the store.

The center aisles of the store are where the processed foods live. The perimeter of the store is where the fruits, vegetables and meats are located. Shopping the edges of the store means that you will fill your cart with healthy foods instead of processed convenience foods that offer little nutritional value. And remember—just because it says "all natural" on the box doesn't mean that it's good for you. Beetles are "all natural"...and ground up beetles are a key ingredient in some "natural" flavors. Yuck.

Cook dinner together with your spouse or significant other.

If you (like me) hate cooking, you are more likely to grab something processed that is easy to prepare, or throw up your hands and go out to eat instead of making meals at home. Grab your spouse, significant other, neighbor, cat...get someone in that kitchen with you. Cooking is more enjoyable when you have a partner and can divide the work while you chat.

Listen to your body.

Just because the clock says that it's dinnertime doesn't mean that you need to sit down to a meal. If you aren't hungry, don't eat. And stop eating when you feel full. Most of us grew up with the "starving children in Africa" mantra chanted religiously at meals. While it is true that there are starving children in Africa, forcing yourself to finish a meal when you are no longer hungry isn't going to change their lives.

Slow down, Harvey!

Bolting your food accomplishes two things. First, it makes you an insufferable bore. And secondly, it can actually cause you to overeat. Your body needs time to get the food that you're eating to your stomach, and then tell your brain that you are full. If you eat like the house is on fire, none of this happens. Your body doesn't know it's full, and you keep eating. Slow down, enjoy your food and give your body a chance to do its' job.

Don't eat late at night.

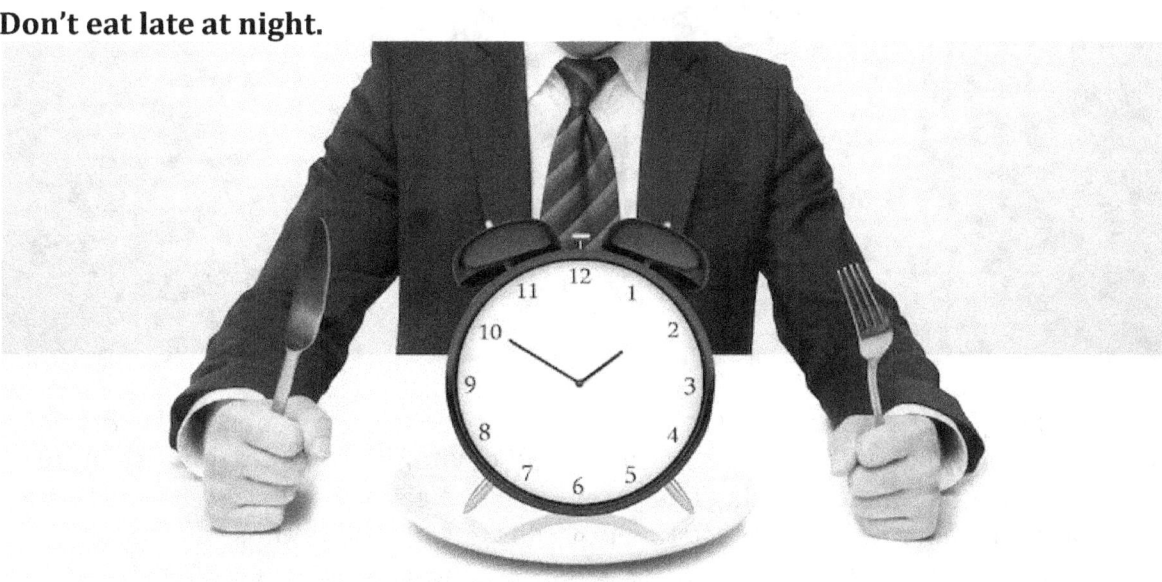

Your body has to work to process the food that you've eaten. If you are eating late at night, the processing is taking place while you are supposed to be sleeping, and you may not sleep as well due to your body not being able to "shut itself off" when it needs to. If you feel like you need something late in the evening, try a banana or a teaspoon of peanut butter. They are easily digested and won't keep you awake.

Quit skipping breakfast.

When you wake up in the morning, your body needs fuel to get started on your day. Skipping breakfast means that you are depriving yourself of the nutrients needed to jump start your day, and you are more likely to grab an unhealthy snack mid-morning or overeat at lunch to make up for the deficit.

Eat the rainbow.

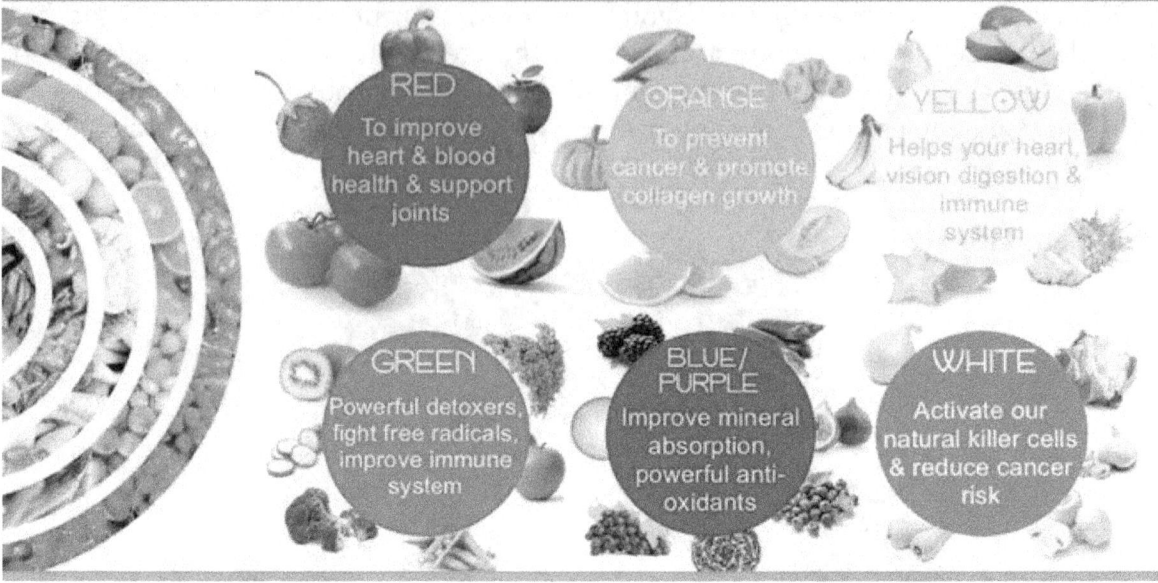

Nature has given us a beautiful array of colors to choose from in our foods. Fruits and vegetables that are brightly colored are full of vitamins and nutrients that are good for our bodies and pleasing to our palates. The general rule is that the brighter the color, the more nutrient-dense the food. So chow down on those cherries, blueberries, dark leafy greens and bright yellow squashes—they are good for you!

Chapter 3: Get up and move it move it!

Physical activity is good for us, body and soul. Our ancestors didn't need to think about exercising because they were moving all day long. Our modern lifestyle means that we sit more and move less and we're feeling the effects of it. The rate of childhood obesity has more than doubled in the past 30 years, and more than two-thirds of adults in the United States are considered overweight or obese. We are literally sitting ourselves to death. Here are some great ideas to get you up and moving!

Take the stairs!

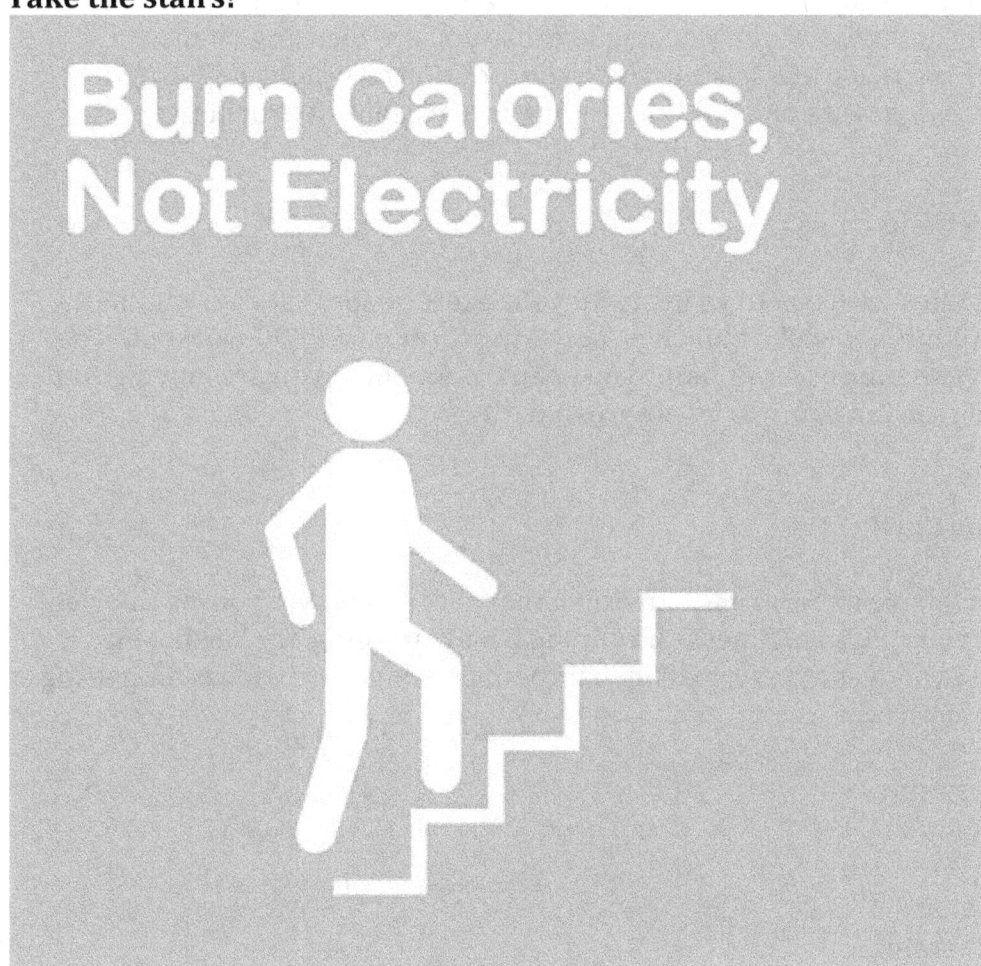

Taking the stairs instead of the elevator can provide a mini-workout and takes just a couple of minutes a day. If you can't take the stairs all the way to your floor, try walking up one floor and then catching the elevator, with the goal of adding a new floor each week. In no time flat you'll be walking all the way up!

Walk, walk, walk.

Whenever you can, walk. If you live in the city and usually take the bus or trolley or subway, try walking to where you're going. If you can't walk all the way, walk a few blocks and then catch your ride. Add a block or two each week until you're up to where you want to be. If you are headed to the mall, park a little farther away than you usually do and walk the extra distance. Take a couple of extra laps around the mall when you are shopping. If you are having a phone conversation, walk around while you're talking. Walk the dog, walk the cat, walk the hamster…pets are a great motivation for movement.

Find a partner.

Grab a girlfriend and go for a walk. As you are walking and chatting, you'll find that you don't really notice what you're doing because you are focusing on the conversation! And if you are starting a workout routine or weight-loss program, find a partner to do it with and hold each other accountable. It provides great motivation!

Keep an exercise journal.

Take a few minutes each day to write down your exercise for that day, whether it was taking a 10-minute walk at lunch or powering through a PX90 workout. The journal serves two purposes—it helps you keep track of how you are moving, and over time you'll see how far you've progressed.

Try something new!

Exercise doesn't have to be boring. Anything that gets you moving burns calories and improves your physical fitness. If running isn't your thing, try kickboxing. If aerobics makes you want to cry, take up ballroom dancing. Some ideas for getting you up and going are…

- Jumping rope
- Dancing
- Boxing
- Bike riding
- Skateboarding
- Rollerblading
- Walking the dog
- Housework (Remember the vacuum scene from "Mrs. Doubtfire"?) Put on some music and clean that house!
- Cut the grass (riding mowers don't count!)
- Rake leaves
- Fly a kite

- Go canoeing
- Swim
- Go golfing (and skip the cart!)
- Ultimate Frisbee

Whatever makes you move—get up and do it! And remember—you may not be moving very fast, but you're moving faster than you were when you were plopped on the couch!

Set goals!

Give yourself something to shoot for. Keep track of your progress in your journal and when you get there, celebrate it big!

Chapter 4: Change the way you think

This one can be tough. Our mind can be our greatest asset and our greatest frustration. Changing the way we think about ourselves takes effort and sometimes it's more difficult than the physical changes that we need to make. It is, however, the best thing that we can do for ourselves. Here are some ways to change your thinking.

Be positive.

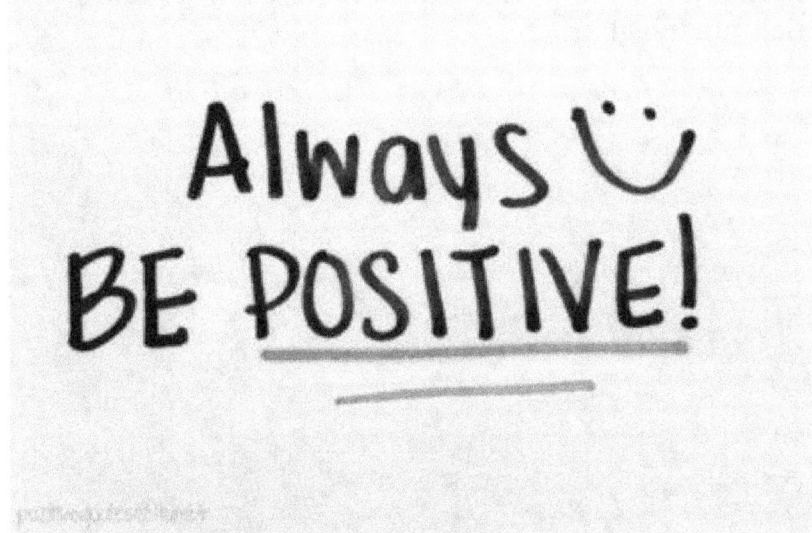

The way we think can affect our performance at our job, how others see us and how we see ourselves. Henry Ford said "Whether you think you can or you think you can't...you're right". Start today to think about yourself in a positive light. Give yourself credit for the things you do well. There is a difference between thinking that we are so amazing that we cross the line into narcissism and being fair and honest about our abilities. Everyone has things that they are good at, and it's time you started recognizing yours.

Keep a "joy journal".

Begin writing down the things that bring you joy every day. They don't have to be big things—waking up in the morning and seeing the sunshine come through the curtains, or hearing the rainfall can bring us joy. A flower, a baby's smile, the smell of coffee drifting through the house...find joy in the little things. And when the joys are big things, celebrate those too! Changing your outlook from negative to positive will go a long way toward changing not only how you feel about yourself, but how you feel about the world in general.

Learn to say "no".

You are not a superhero. You cannot do everything that everyone asks of you, no matter how hard you try, and if you find that you are neglecting yourself or your family because you are so overcommitted, it's time to say "no". Your worth is not measured by how much you can "do", and setting limits on your time, your commitments and your talents is not being selfish.

Find your words.

Collect quotes, affirmations, words of encouragement. Write them down on notecards and put them in strategic places where you will see them. Keep a journal in your purse, car, desk...anywhere that you are. Write down the words that encourage and inspire you and refer back to them when you need a pick-me-up. Words have great power, both to hurt and to heal. Keep the ones that heal and discard the rest. Remember—just because it was said doesn't mean it was true.

Chapter 5: Think outside your box

It is easy to get into a rut and just do the same thing, over and over. Living an active, healthy lifestyle involves constantly improving ourselves physically, mentally and spiritually. You are never too old to learn something new. You are never too busy to give of your time and talents (but remember—say "no" when you need to!) and even if you have next to nothing, you still have yourself. And giving of ourselves is often the most precious gift anyone can receive. Here are some ideas for thinking "outside the box"…

Volunteer.

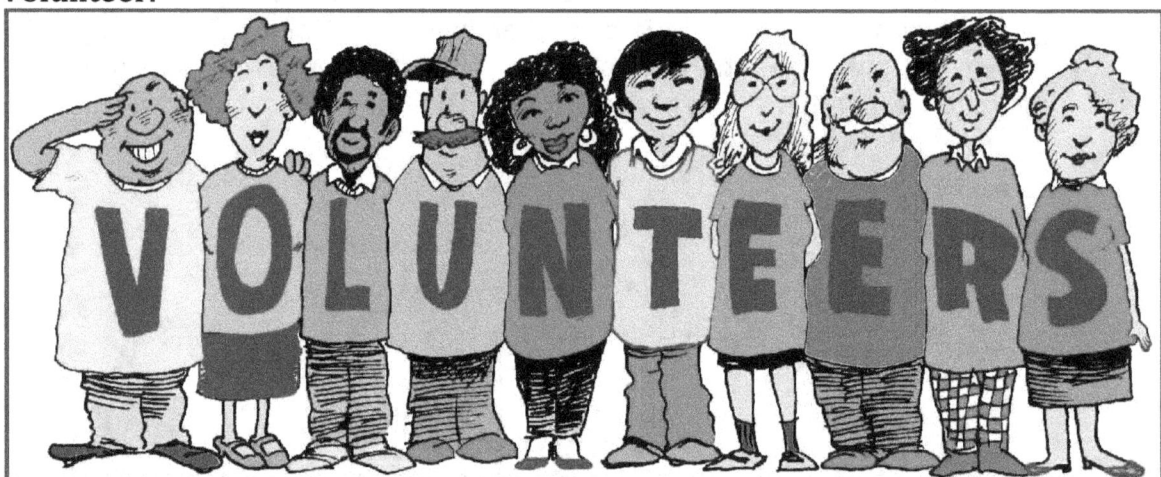

It doesn't cost any money to volunteer. Taking even an hour out of your busy schedule to do something for someone else will make you feel better, even if your own circumstances are less than ideal. Some ideas for volunteering include:

- Serving a meal at a soup kitchen
- Helping a housebound neighbor with errands
- Working in the nursery at church once a month
- Watching a friend's children so that she can get out on a date with her husband
- Volunteering to help plant or care for a community garden
- Working as a trail guide in a national park
- Rocking babies at a local hospital
- Volunteering at a local animal shelter
- Helping in your child's classroom at school

These are just a few ideas to help you get started. The possibilities are endless, and don't have to be local. If you have a little more time, consider taking a missions trip, either somewhere in the US or overseas, to help with projects that will improve the lives of people who truly have nothing.

Learn something new.

Even if you graduated from high school back during the Lincoln administration, you're still here and you are still capable of learning something new! Take a cooking class, learn to paint, write a book...harness your creativity and learn to do something new, just because you've always wanted to. Give yourself permission to spend an hour a week on yourself and tackle something that you've always wanted to do and never had "time" for. Take singing lessons. Learn to play the tuba. Take a class on flower arranging. Learn to sew and make yourself a new wardrobe. Learn a new language and then take a trip and use it! It doesn't have to make sense, and no one has to understand why you're doing it except you.

Find your passion.

"Don't ask what the world needs. Ask what makes you come alive, and go do it. Because what the world needs are people who have come alive." — Howard Thurman

We all have a passion. Something that lights our fire, makes our eyes sparkle, makes us passionately angry, and makes us passionately alive. Take time to talk to yourself. Ask yourself when you are the most alive. It may have been twenty years ago when you were a carefree college student dedicated to changing the world. It may be now, in a house full of toddlers and diapers and Cheerios. Maybe you feel most alive when you are helping someone. Or inventing something that will make someone's life better.

Maybe, like me, your passion lies in words. Start writing. Even if no one but you ever reads them, your words are yours alone and they have the power to inspire you. Perhaps you are passionate about the injustice in the world. You may never change the entire world, but you can make a difference right where you are. Learn what you can and educate people about the issues that matter most to you.

Chapter 6: Random habits for a better you

Sometimes things don't fit into neat little boxes and neither should you. You are unique. There is only one you and you have talents and abilities that no one else has. It's time to look at yourself from a realistic perspective and start adopting healthy habits that will make you a better person, both inside and out. You are never too old to improve. Remember...

"Life should not be a journey to the grave with the intention of arriving safely in a pretty and well preserved body, but rather to skid in broadside in a cloud of smoke, thoroughly used up, totally worn out, and loudly proclaiming "Wow! What a Ride!" — Hunter S. Thompson

Turn off the TV.

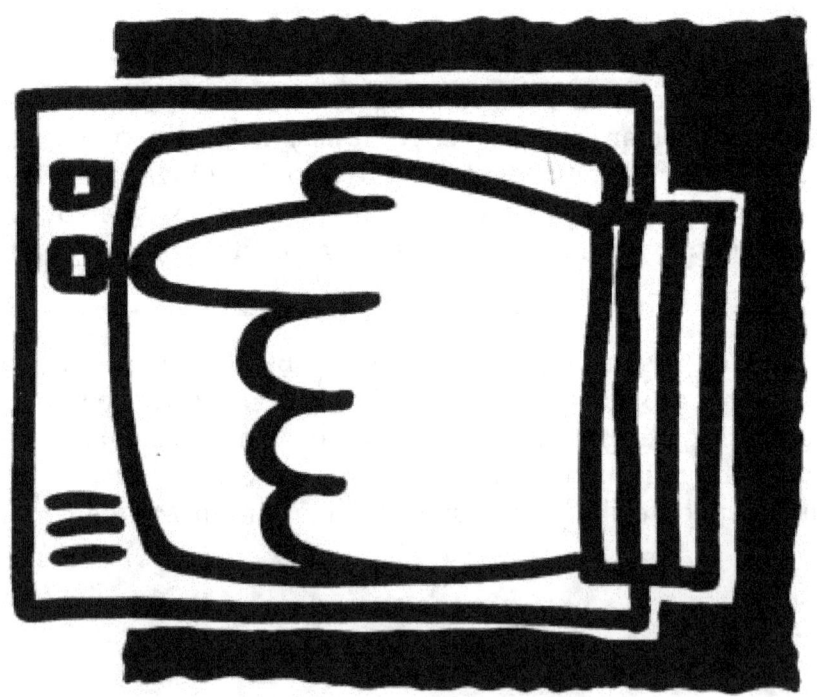

Turn off TV.
Turn on life

A little is fine, but too much TV is just not good for anyone. Even watching the news exposes us to the negativity that permeates our world, and can cause us to develop negative thinking patterns. While it is important to know what is happening in the world, don't allow yourself to become obsessed with it. Take the time to see the good in the world too, and whenever possible, focus on that.

Be thankful.

Be intentionally thankful for your life. You have a lot to be thankful for, whether you are ready to admit it or not. Think about it…

- **You can read**. Over 774 million adults on this planet cannot say the same thing, and more than 72 million children lack access to even the most basic of educations.
- **You are free to read what you want to**. Millions of people across the planet are forbidden to read anything except what their government deems "acceptable".
- **You have access to a computer**. Even in our increasingly technological world, there are millions of people who do not have access to the tools to help them compete in the global playing field.
- **You likely have some loose change in your pocket, lying around the house, in the cup holder between the seats of your car**. This puts you in the top 8% of the world's wealthiest people. More than 2 billion people subsist on less than $1 a day.
- **You are free to worship as you please**. In the United States, we are guaranteed the right to worship the way we choose, without fear of reprisal. Millions of people across the globe cannot claim that right, and hundreds will die for their faith just in the time it takes you to read this.

- **You have access to medical care**. 21 children die every minute from preventable diseases. In the time it's taken you to read this short book, hundreds of children have died from things that could have been stopped with simple medical care.

Assume that people have good intentions.

In today's world, where the news is filled with story after story of violence and evil, it can be easy to become cynical and angry. Make a conscious effort to assume the good in people. Finding the good in other people will help you to see the good in yourself.

Learn to forgive.

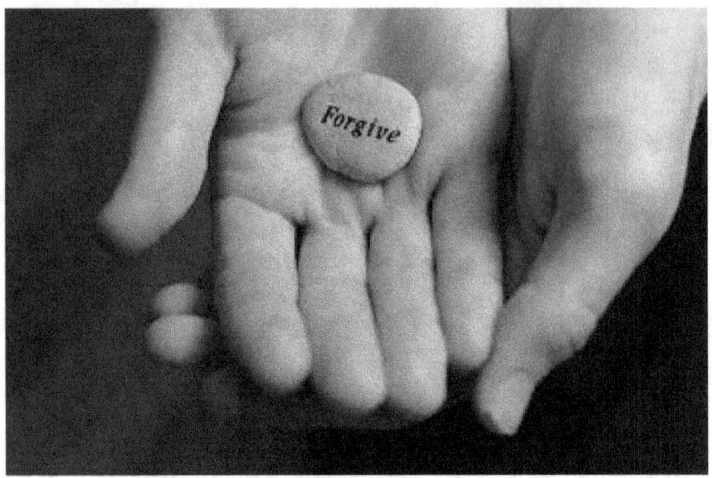

Someone once said that "holding a grudge is kind of like drinking poison and waiting for the other person to die". Meanwhile, the person who is slowly dying is you. Learn to cultivate an attitude of forgiveness. Doing so can have physiological benefits such as lower blood pressure, less stress and quicker recovery from trauma, and it also has emotional benefits. By releasing the stress associated with holding a grudge, you are freeing your mind and your emotions to go to a place of positivity.

Spend time with your friends.

Even introverts need a social network. Spending time with friends and family boosts your self-esteem and even helps you to feel better physically. And having a deep connection to others allows you to see yourself through their eyes and put things in a more positive light.

Give yourself permission to express your emotions.
Allow yourself to laugh, cry, grow angry, and feel pain. Suppressing emotions leads to physical problems such as heart issues and high blood pressure, and creates emotional walls that can be difficult to tear down. Even anger can be expressed appropriately, and learning to express your feelings and emotions is part of being a healthy, well-balanced adult.

Conclusion

Cultivating a healthy lifestyle means building on a foundation of good habits. You don't have to jump in and implement every single suggestion that we've given you here in one fell swoop (in fact, we strongly recommend that you don't) but taking time to look at your life in an honest and non-judgmental way, then deciding what areas need improvement will go a long way toward living a healthier, happier life.

You are not powerless to change your life. In fact, you are holding all the keys to what you need. Only you can summon up the motivation to make the changes that need to be changed. You are the master of your thought life—no one else can change your thoughts and attitudes for you. While therapy can be beneficial in helping you to recognize areas that need improvement, when it comes down to the wire, you are the one who has to make the final call.

Any time you make changes in your life; there is a certain amount of fear involved. Asking yourself some simple questions can help to guide you as you begin to implement changes...

- Will this help me to feel better (spiritually, mentally, physically)
- What will happen if I don't make the change (stagnating, poor health)
- Can I trust myself to know what is best for me?

When you begin to implement change in your life, start by setting realistic goals. If you need to lose 100 pounds and haven't exercised since the 5th grade, then setting a goal of running five miles a day and losing all of the weight in three months is not realistic. Give yourself room to grow. Once you have met your goals, look back and see what helped you achieve them, and what might have hindered you, and then set new goals based on what you learned. Celebrate your victories—you worked hard to get where you are, and even if it's not where you plan to end up, you are that much closer to where you want to be!

"You're off to Great Places!
Today is your day!
Your mountain is waiting,
So... get on your way!" — Dr. Seuss